ADHD MANAGEMENT FOR KIDS

Understanding Your Child's ADHD: A Parent's Guide to Managing Symptoms

LAUREN M. GREEN

Copyright

Published by [Lauren M. Green], [2023].

TABLE OF CONTENTS

Chapter one

Chapter Two

Chapter Three

Chapter Four

Chapter Five

Chapter Six

INTRODUCTION

Attention Deficit Hyperactivity Disorder (ADHD) is a neurodevelopmental disorder that affects children and often continues into adulthood. It is characterized by symptoms such as inattention, hyperactivity, and impulsivity that can interfere with a child's daily functioning and social interactions.

Managing ADHD in children involves a comprehensive approach that includes various strategies, such as behavioral interventions, medication, and parental support. The goal of treatment is to improve a child's ability to focus, control their impulses, and manage their behavior in different settings such as at school and at home.

Behavioral interventions involve teaching children skills to manage their symptoms, such as improving their organizational skills, time management, and social skills. Medication can also be used to help manage symptoms. Stimulant medications, such as methylphenidate (Ritalin) and amphetamine (Adderall), are the most commonly prescribed medications for ADHD.

Parental support is also an important part of managing ADHD in children. Parents can help their children by creating a structured environment, establishing consistent routines, and providing positive reinforcement for desired behaviors.

Overall, managing ADHD in children requires a collaborative effort between parents, teachers, healthcare providers, and other caregivers to ensure that children with ADHD receive the appropriate support and care to reach their full potential.

Chapter one

Explanation of ADHD in children

ADHD is a neurodevelopmental disorder that affects children and can continue into adulthood. It is characterized by symptoms of inattention, hyperactivity, and impulsivity that can impact a child's daily functioning and social interactions.

Inattention symptoms can include difficulty paying attention or focusing on tasks, forgetfulness, and being easily distracted. Hyperactivity symptoms can include excessive fidgeting or restlessness, difficulty sitting still, and excessive talking. Impulsivity symptoms can include interrupting others, acting without thinking, and difficulty waiting their turn.

ADHD can affect a child's academic performance, social relationships, and self-esteem. Children with ADHD may struggle with completing tasks, following instructions, and staying organized. They may also have trouble with making friends or engaging in appropriate social behavior.

The exact causes of ADHD are not fully understood, but it is believed to be caused by a combination of genetic, environmental, and developmental factors. Some risk factors for ADHD include a family history of ADHD, premature birth or low birth weight, exposure to toxins, and maternal smoking or alcohol use during pregnancy.

ADHD is typically diagnosed by a healthcare professional, such as a pediatrician or psychiatrist, who will evaluate a child's symptoms and may conduct psychological testing. Treatment for ADHD typically involves a combination of behavioral interventions, medication, and parental support. With appropriate management and support, children with ADHD can learn to manage their symptoms and thrive.

Prevalence of ADHD

ADHD is a relatively common neurodevelopmental disorder that affects children and adults worldwide. According to the Centers for Disease Control and Prevention (CDC), the prevalence of ADHD in children in the United States is estimated to be around 9.4%. This means that about 1 in 11 children in the United States have ADHD.

ADHD affects boys more commonly than girls, with boys being diagnosed with ADHD about three times as often as girls. However, this difference may be due in part to.

differences in how boys and girls exhibit ADHD symptoms, with boys more likely to display hyperactivity symptoms and girls more likely to display inattention symptoms.

The prevalence of ADHD varies across different countries and cultures. Studies have shown that ADHD is more commonly diagnosed in Western countries than in non-Western countries. However, this may be due in part to differences in diagnostic criteria and cultural attitudes towards ADHD.

Overall, ADHD is a significant public health concern that can impact a child's academic performance, social relationships, and overall quality of life. Early diagnosis and appropriate management can help children with ADHD learn to manage their symptoms and thrive.

Importance of ADHD management

ADHD management is important because it can help children with ADHD learn to manage their symptoms and improve their overall functioning and quality of life. ADHD can impact a child's academic performance, social relationships, and self-esteem, but with appropriate management, children with ADHD can learn to overcome these challenges and reach their full potential.

Untreated ADHD can have negative consequences for a child's development and future outcomes. Children with untreated ADHD are at an increased risk for academic difficulties, behavioral problems, substance abuse, and mental health issues later in life.

Effective ADHD management involves a combination of behavioral interventions, medication, and parental support. Behavioral interventions, such as cognitive-behavioral therapy and parent training, can help children learn skills to manage their symptoms and improve their academic and social functioning. Medication, such as stimulant medications, can also be effective in managing ADHD symptoms.

Parental support is also an important component of ADHD management. Parents can help their children with ADHD by creating a structured environment, establishing consistent routines, and providing positive reinforcement for desired behaviors.

Overall, managing ADHD in children is important for their well-being and future outcomes. With appropriate management and support, children with ADHD can learn to manage their symptoms and thrive.

Chapter Two

Overview of ADHD symptoms in children

Attention-deficit/hyperactivity disorder (ADHD) is a neurodevelopmental disorder that affects children's ability to focus, control their impulses, and regulate their behavior. Children with ADHD may struggle with academic performance, social relationships, and self-esteem.

The symptoms of ADHD can vary from child to child but generally fall into two categories: inattention and hyperactivity/impulsivity. Inattention symptoms can include difficulty paying attention or focusing, forgetfulness, and being easily distracted. Hyperactivity/impulsivity symptoms can include restlessness, fidgeting, interrupting others, and acting without thinking.

There are different types of ADHD recognized by healthcare professionals, including predominantly inattentive type, predominantly hyperactive-impulsive type, and combined type. Proper diagnosis and classification of ADHD type is important for appropriate management and treatment.

It's important to note that these symptoms can also be present in children without ADHD, so a proper diagnosis by a healthcare professional is necessary. Additionally, symptoms may change or manifest differently as a child ages and develops.

Overall, understanding the symptoms of ADHD is important for early identification and appropriate management. With proper diagnosis and treatment, children with

ADHD can learn to manage their symptoms and thrive.

Different types of ADHD

There are three different types of ADHD recognized by the Diagnostic and Statistical Manual of Mental Disorders (DSM-5), which is the standard classification system used by healthcare professionals to diagnose mental health conditions. These types are:

Inattention symptoms of ADHD in children can include:

- Difficulty paying attention or focusing on tasks, such as schoolwork or homework
- Making careless mistakes on assignments or activities
- Struggling to follow instructions or complete tasks

- Difficulty organizing tasks or belongings
- Avoiding or disliking tasks that require sustained mental effort
- Frequently losing or misplacing items
- Easily distracted by external stimuli
- Forgetfulness and absent-mindedness

Hyperactivity/impulsivity symptoms of ADHD in children can include:

- Fidgeting or squirming in their seats
- Difficulty sitting still or staying seated in appropriate situations
- Constantly "on the go" or seeming to be driven by a motor
- Talking excessively, interrupting others, or blurting out answers before the question has been completed
- Difficulty waiting their turn or taking turns in conversations or games

- Intruding on others' conversations or activities
- Impatience and difficulty delaying gratification

Combined Type: This is the most common type of ADHD and is characterized by symptoms of both inattention and hyperactivity/impulsivity. Children with this type of ADHD display symptoms of both inattention and hyperactivity/impulsivity.

It's important to note that the DSM-5 diagnostic criteria for ADHD require the presence of symptoms that impair daily functioning and are not attributable to another medical or psychiatric condition. Additionally, symptoms can vary in severity and may change or manifest differently as a child ages and develops.

Criteria for ADHD diagnosis

The American Psychiatric Association's Diagnostic and Statistical Manual of Mental Disorders (DSM-5) outlines the following criteria for the diagnosis of ADHD:

1. **Inattention:** The individual must display at least six symptoms of inattention, such as difficulty sustaining attention in tasks, making careless mistakes, forgetting things necessary for tasks, losing things necessary for tasks, easily distracted by external stimuli, and difficulty organizing tasks and activities.

2. **Hyperactivity/Impulsivity:** The individual must display at least six symptoms of hyperactivity and/or impulsivity, such as fidgeting or squirming, difficulty remaining seated, excessive talking, interrupting others,

difficulty waiting their turn, and acting without thinking.

3. **Onset and Duration:** The individual must display several of these symptoms before the age of 12, and the symptoms must be present in two or more settings (e.g., home, school, social situations). The symptoms must also be present for at least six months and interfere with daily functioning.

4. **Severity:** The symptoms must be severe enough to cause significant impairment in academic, social, or occupational functioning.

5. **Exclusionary Criteria:** The symptoms cannot be better explained by another mental disorder, such as anxiety or depression, and cannot be attributable to another medical condition, medication use, or substance abuse.

It's important to note that the diagnosis of ADHD requires a comprehensive evaluation that includes a detailed medical and family history, a physical exam, and assessment of symptoms. The evaluation may also include input from teachers and other caregivers.

It's recommended that the diagnosis of ADHD be made by a qualified healthcare professional with expertise in ADHD, such as a pediatrician, psychiatrist, or psychologist.

Chapter Three

Treatment Options for ADHD Kids

There are several treatment options available to help manage these symptoms and improve a child's quality of life. In this response, we will explore some of the different treatment options available for ADHD in children, including medication, behavioral interventions and combined therapy . It is important for parents to work closely with their child's healthcare provider to determine the best treatment plan for their child's individual needs.

Medication management for ADHD

Medication management is a common treatment approach for individuals with Attention Deficit Hyperactivity Disorder (ADHD). There are two main types of medications used to treat ADHD: stimulants and non-stimulants.

Stimulant medications are the most commonly prescribed medications for ADHD. They work by increasing the levels of dopamine and norepinephrine in the brain, which can improve attention, focus, and impulse control. Examples of stimulant medications include methylphenidate (Ritalin, Concerta, Metadate) and amphetamines (Adderall, Dexedrine).

Non-stimulant medications are another option for individuals with ADHD who may not respond well to stimulant medications or have certain medical conditions that make stimulants less appropriate. Non-stimulant medications work by increasing the levels of norepinephrine in the brain. Examples of non-stimulant medications include atomoxetine (Strattera), guanfacine (Intuniv), and clonidine (Kapvay).

It is important to work with a healthcare provider to determine the best medication and dosage for the individual with ADHD. The medication should be monitored regularly to ensure it is effective and not causing any adverse side effects. Other non-medication strategies, such as behavioral therapy and lifestyle changes, can also be incorporated into the treatment plan to help manage symptoms of ADHD.

Behavioral interventions for ADHD

Behavioral interventions are an important component of the treatment plan for children with Attention Deficit Hyperactivity Disorder (ADHD). These interventions focus on teaching children new skills and behaviors to help them manage their symptoms and improve their social and academic functioning. Some examples of behavioral interventions for ADHD include:

Behavioral therapy: This type of therapy teaches children new coping strategies, such as organizational skills and time management techniques, to help them better manage their ADHD symptoms. Behavioral therapy may be delivered through individual, group, or family sessions.

Parent training: Parents of children with ADHD can benefit from training on behavior management techniques to help them better support their child at home. This may include teaching parents how to provide positive reinforcement for good behavior and set clear rules and consequences for negative behavior.

Social skills training: Children with ADHD may struggle with social interactions and making and maintaining friendships. Social skills training can teach children the necessary skills to navigate social situations and develop positive relationships with their peers.

Classroom accommodations: Teachers can make accommodations in the classroom to help children with ADHD stay focused and engaged. This may include preferential seating, reduced distractions, and breaking down tasks into smaller, manageable steps.

Organizational skills training: Children with ADHD often struggle with organization, which can impact their academic performance. Organizational skills training can teach children how to effectively manage their time, plan and prioritize tasks, and keep track of assignments and deadlines.

Behavioral interventions are often used in combination with medication to provide comprehensive treatment for children with ADHD.

Combination therapy

Combination therapy, which involves the use of both medication and behavioral interventions, is often the most effective approach for treating children with Attention Deficit Hyperactivity Disorder (ADHD).

Medications such as stimulants and non-stimulants can help manage the core symptoms of ADHD, such as inattention, hyperactivity, and impulsivity. However, medication alone may not be enough to address all of the challenges that children with ADHD face.

Behavioral interventions, such as behavioral therapy, parent training, social skills training, and organizational skills training, can help children with ADHD learn new skills and behaviors to manage their symptoms and improve their social and academic functioning.

Combining medication and behavioral interventions can provide a more comprehensive approach to treating ADHD. For example, medication may help improve a child's ability to focus and stay on task, while behavioral interventions can teach them skills to manage their time, stay organized, and cope with stress.

Chapter Four

Parental Support

Strategies for parents to support their children with ADHD

Parents play a crucial role in supporting their children with Attention Deficit Hyperactivity Disorder (ADHD). Here are some strategies that parents can use to support their child with ADHD:

Education: Parents should learn as much as they can about ADHD, including its symptoms, causes, and treatment options. This can help them better understand their child's condition and how to support them.

Structure and Routine: Children with ADHD benefit from structure and routine.

Parents can create a consistent schedule for their child that includes designated times for meals, homework, and other activities.

Positive reinforcement: Praising and rewarding children for good behavior can help reinforce positive behaviors and improve their self-esteem. Parents should focus on praising their child's efforts and progress, rather than only focusing on their mistakes.

Clear expectations: Children with ADHD may struggle with understanding what is expected of them. Parents can make expectations clear by breaking tasks into smaller, manageable steps and giving clear instructions.

Organization: Children with ADHD often struggle with organization. Parents can help their child stay organized by creating a designated study area, using checklists or visual aids, and helping them break down tasks into smaller steps.

Open communication: Parents should maintain open communication with their child's healthcare provider, teacher, and other professionals involved in their care. This can help ensure that their child is receiving the appropriate support and treatment.

Self-care: Parenting a child with ADHD can be challenging and stressful. Parents should prioritize their own self-care and seek support when needed, such as through a support group or therapy.

These strategies can help parents better support their child with ADHD and improve their child's overall well-being.

Importance of open communication with healthcare providers

Open communication with healthcare providers is especially important for children with ADHD (Attention-Deficit/Hyperactivity Disorder) and their families. Here are some of the key reasons why:

Accurate diagnosis: Open communication with healthcare providers can help ensure that children with ADHD receive an accurate diagnosis. Parents can provide important information about their child's behavior and symptoms, which can help healthcare providers make a proper diagnosis and create an effective treatment plan.

Tailored treatment: Open communication can help healthcare providers tailor treatment plans to meet the specific needs of each child with ADHD. Parents can discuss their child's preferences and concerns, and healthcare providers can adjust treatment strategies accordingly.

Medication management: Children with ADHD may be prescribed medication to help manage their symptoms. Open communication can help ensure that medication is prescribed and administered correctly, and that any potential side effects are monitored.

Behavioral interventions: Behavioral interventions, such as therapy and parent training, can also be effective in managing ADHD symptoms. Open communication can help parents and healthcare providers work together to identify and implement appropriate interventions.

Support for families: Open communication can help families of children with ADHD feel supported and informed. Healthcare providers can provide guidance on managing ADHD symptoms, accessing resources and support groups, and coping with the challenges of raising a child with ADHD.

In summary, open communication with healthcare providers is critical for ensuring that children with ADHD receive accurate diagnoses, tailored treatment plans, and effective support. Parents should feel comfortable discussing their concerns, asking questions, and providing honest information about their child's behavior and symptoms.

Addressing challenges with school and social interactions

Children with Attention-Deficit/Hyperactivity Disorder (ADHD) may face challenges with school and social interactions. Here are some strategies to address these challenges:

School challenges:

Communicate with your child's teacher: Discuss your child's needs and work together to develop a plan that supports their learning. This may include accommodations such as extra time on tests or breaks during class.

Break tasks into smaller steps: Children with ADHD may struggle with tasks that require sustained attention. Breaking tasks into smaller steps can make them more manageable.

Use visual aids: Visual aids, such as checklists or schedules, can help children with ADHD stay organized and on-task.

Social interactions:

Teach social skills: Children with ADHD may struggle with social skills such as taking turns, listening, and staying on topic. Social skills training can help them develop these skills.

Encourage positive social interactions: Praise your child when they engage in positive social interactions such as sharing or cooperating.

Provide opportunities for socialization: Encourage your child to participate in activities that allow them to interact with peers who share their interests.

Overall support:

Maintain a routine: Children with ADHD may benefit from a structured routine that includes regular sleep, meals, and homework time.

Use positive reinforcement: Reward your child for positive behavior rather than focusing on negative behavior.

Seek support: Consider joining a support group for parents of children with ADHD or seeking the help of a mental health professional.

In summary, addressing challenges with school and social interactions for children with ADHD may involve working with teachers, breaking tasks into smaller steps, using visual aids, teaching social skills, providing opportunities for socialization, maintaining a routine, using positive reinforcement, and seeking support.

Chapter Five

Accommodations and modifications for children with ADHD in the classroom

Attention-deficit/hyperactivity disorder (ADHD) can affect a child's ability to focus, pay attention, and follow instructions in the classroom. Therefore, it is essential to make accommodations and modifications to help these students succeed academically and socially.

Here are some possible strategies:

Provide a structured environment: Children with ADHD often benefit from a predictable routine, so establish clear expectations, rules, and schedules. Use visual aids such as calendars, timers, and checklists to help them stay on task.

Reduce distractions: Minimize potential distractions in the classroom by seating the student away from windows, doors, and other sources of noise or movement. Consider using noise-canceling headphones or white noise machines to create a quieter environment.

Use multisensory learning: Engage the student with ADHD by providing hands-on activities, using visuals, and incorporating movement into the lesson. Allow them to stand or pace while working on a task.

Break down complex tasks: Divide complex assignments or projects into smaller, manageable parts. Provide step-by-step instructions, and check in frequently to make sure the student understands what they need to do.

Provide frequent feedback: Children with ADHD often benefit from immediate feedback on their work. Use positive reinforcement, such as verbal praise or stickers, to encourage good behavior and effort.

Allow for movement breaks: Provide opportunities for the student to move around and take breaks, such as going for a short walk or doing some stretching exercises.

Adjust workload and expectations: Adjust the workload and expectations based on the student's ability level. Set realistic goals and celebrate small accomplishments to build confidence.

Communicate with parents and other professionals: Work closely with parents, counselors, and other professionals to develop a comprehensive plan for supporting the student with ADHD. Regularly communicate with them to monitor progress and make adjustments as needed.

Remember that accommodations and modifications may vary depending on the individual needs of each student with ADHD. Consult with your school's special education team or seek the advice of a licensed healthcare professional for further guidance.

Collaboration with school professionals for kids with ADHD

Collaboration with school professionals is an essential aspect of supporting kids with ADHD. By working together, parents, teachers, and other school professionals can develop effective strategies and accommodations that can help these children succeed in school. Here are some tips for collaborating with school professionals for kids with ADHD:

Establish open communication: Make sure that lines of communication are open between you, your child's teacher, and any other school professionals involved in your child's education. This may include the school psychologist, special education teacher, or guidance counselor.

Share information about your child: Share information about your child's ADHD diagnosis, treatment, and any specific concerns or challenges that you have noticed at home. This can help school professionals understand your child's needs better and develop appropriate strategies and accommodations.

Work together to create an individualized education plan (IEP) or 504 plan: If your child has been diagnosed with ADHD, they may be eligible for an IEP or 504 plan. These plans outline specific accommodations and strategies that can help your child succeed in school. Work with school professionals to create an individualized plan that meets your child's needs.

Monitor progress: Regularly monitor your child's progress and discuss any concerns or successes with school professionals. This can help ensure that the strategies and accommodations being used are effective and make any necessary adjustments.

Advocate for your child: If you feel that your child is not receiving appropriate support or accommodations, speak up and advocate for your child's needs. Remember that you are your child's best advocate and partner with school professionals to ensure that your child is getting the support they need to succeed in school.

Chapter Six

Healthy lifestyle habits to support ADHD management

There are several healthy lifestyle habits that can help support the management of ADHD in children:

Regular Exercise: Physical activity can help improve attention, reduce hyperactivity and impulsivity, and improve overall mood. Encouraging children to engage in regular physical activity, such as playing outside, sports, or dancing, can be helpful.

Balanced Diet: Providing children with a balanced diet that includes plenty of fruits and vegetables, whole grains, lean protein, and healthy fats can help improve concentration and energy levels. Avoiding sugary and processed foods can also be helpful.

Consistent Sleep Routine: Children with ADHD often struggle with sleep, so establishing a consistent bedtime routine that includes calming activities before bed can be helpful. It is recommended that children get between 9-11 hours of sleep each night.

Mindfulness Techniques: Teaching children mindfulness techniques such as deep breathing, yoga, or meditation can help them learn to focus their attention and regulate their emotions.

Positive Reinforcement: Praising children for positive behavior and accomplishments, rather than focusing solely on negative behaviors, can help improve their self-esteem and motivation.

Organizational Support: Children with ADHD may need help staying organized, so providing them with tools such as a planner or visual schedule can be helpful. Additionally, breaking tasks into smaller steps can make them feel more manageable.

Medication Management: For some children with ADHD, medication may be recommended as part of their treatment plan. It is important to work closely with a healthcare provider to ensure that medications are being used safely and effectively.

Overall, incorporating healthy lifestyle habits into a child's routine can help support the management of ADHD. By focusing on regular exercise, a balanced diet, consistent sleep routines, mindfulness techniques, positive reinforcement, organizational support, and medication management,

parents and caregivers can help children with
ADHD reach their full potential.

**Practical tips for children with ADHD to
succeed at school and at home**

Here are some practical tips for children with
ADHD to succeed at school and at home:

- Establish a routine: Children with
  ADHD thrive on routine and structure.
  Establish a consistent schedule for
  waking up, going to bed, meal times,
  and homework time.

- Create a calm environment: Reduce
  distractions in the home and in the
  child's study area. Provide a quiet place
  for homework and minimize
  background noise.

- Break tasks into smaller chunks: Large tasks can be overwhelming for children with ADHD. Break tasks into smaller, more manageable chunks and provide frequent breaks to help them stay focused.

- Use visual aids: Visual aids such as charts, diagrams, and pictures can help children with ADHD understand and remember information.

- Provide positive reinforcement: Children with ADHD respond well to positive reinforcement. Praise their efforts and accomplishments, and focus on their strengths.

- Encourage physical activity: Exercise can help children with ADHD improve their focus and attention. Encourage regular physical activity, such as outdoor play, sports, or dance.

- Use technology: There are many apps and tools available that can help children with ADHD stay organized and focused. Explore options for time management, organization, and study aids.

- Communicate with teachers: Work with your child's teachers to establish a plan for support and accommodations in the classroom. Keep open lines of communication and work together to find strategies that work for your child.

- Seek professional help: If your child is struggling with ADHD, seek professional help from a mental health professional. They can help provide support and strategies for managing symptoms at home and at school.

- Provide opportunities for self-reflection: Encourage your child to think about their own behavior and how it affects others. Help them identify their strengths and weaknesses, and talk about how they can use their strengths to overcome their challenges.

- Teach self-advocacy skills: Help your child learn how to communicate their needs and preferences to others. This may involve practicing assertiveness and learning how to ask for help when needed.

Hope for positive outcomes with ADHD management.

There is certainly hope for positive outcomes with ADHD management. With proper support, individuals with ADHD can learn to manage their symptoms and lead successful, fulfilling lives. Here are some positive outcomes that are possible with effective ADHD management:

Improved academic and occupational performance: With the right support, individuals with ADHD can improve their focus, organization, and time management skills, leading to better academic and occupational performance.

Better social relationships: ADHD management can help individuals improve their social skills and communication, leading to better relationships with family, friends, and colleagues.

Improved self-esteem and confidence: As individuals learn to manage their symptoms and achieve their goals, their self-esteem and confidence can improve.

Better physical health: With improved self-awareness and self-control, individuals with ADHD can learn to make healthier choices and improve their overall physical health.

Increased independence and autonomy: With appropriate support, individuals with ADHD can learn to manage their symptoms and take responsibility for their own lives, leading to increased independence and autonomy.

Reduced risk of comorbidities: Effective ADHD management can reduce the risk of developing comorbidities such as anxiety and depression, which can occur when ADHD symptoms go unaddressed.

It's important to note that ADHD management is a lifelong process that requires ongoing support and effort. However, with the right support and resources, individuals with ADHD can achieve positive outcomes and lead fulfilling lives.